Weight Management approach Permanent techniques

How to Slim Down for the last time

by

Sandra R. Trimble

TABLE OF CONTENT

INTRODUCTION

Energy intake exceeds metabolic rate, which is the basic foundation for weight gain. However, genetic, behavioral, and environmental factors interact in a complicated manner to cause overweight and obesity. While hundreds, if not thousands, of weight-loss programs, diets, remedies, and devices have been made available to the overweight public. It is difficult for practitioners, researchers, and even the overweight themselves to find long-lasting, efficient programs for weight loss and maintenance due to the multifactorial aetiology of overweight. According to estimates, only 1 to 3 percent of people who successfully lose weight are able to keep it off.

The evidence suggests that genetics may play a role in the development of overweight and obesity, The rise in overweight that has been seen in the population in the last 20 years, however, cannot be attributed to heredity.

Instead, the majority of the blame must go to the psychological and social factors that work together to persuade people to participate in insufficient aerobic fitness and consume excessive amounts of food compared to their metabolic rate. The above elements are the focus of weight-management techniques.

This section of the book examines the effectiveness and stability of weight reduction techniques in addition to the mixtures of techniques that are linked to healthy weight loss. Additionally, as the problem of weight management may lead to an overweight situation, the components of effective weight maintenance will also be examined. There is also a short conversation about public policy initiatives that could effectively deter overweight and support individuals who seek to lose weight or keep it off.

Chapter 1

How to Assess Physical and Emotional Hungry

It's difficult to resist drooling when a commercial for a luscious bacon cheeseburger plays. Or you may keep telling yourself you don't need any more (or more than three) of the delectable chocolate treats while thinking about the pastries you have stashed away.

Are you still famished?

It might be quite difficult to tell when you're genuinely hungry and when your thoughts are just tricking you. People have traditionally struggled with food temptations; these days, it's even more difficult to resist such strong cravings since we can easily order pizza or chicken wings as takeout using mobile applications. Being cooped up inside the house also entails having constant access to the items in our freezers and closets. Although your body is a very adept communicator, it can be easy to misunderstand its signs.

That is true because there could be a thin line separating "that feels extremely wonderful" from "I want food for energy."

"When you factor in things like fatigue and anxiety, it becomes much harder to distinguish between hunger and fullness."

To maintain a healthy weight, an important skill is needed, and caring for your body means learning how to distinguish between being truly hungry and succumbing to a typical eating trigger. To help you eat healthier, here's how to fully understand your body's food cravings.

☐ **Individual But Predictable Hunger Cues**

Hunger is highly individual, just like other health-related issues. As the experiment shows, "two people can consume the same food, with one person still unsatisfied and the other perfectly full."

Regardless of whether you worked out at home at that moment or spent the entire day binge-watching police publications, your dietary demands can also change throughout the day.

The trick is to pay attention to your body's signals and make an effort to understand them.

Keeping a food journal is one approach to achieving this. You'll be forced to identify your eating habits, both good and bad. You might notice, for instance, that you always go for a bag of chocolates to cheer you up in the afternoon or that you always order pizza for movie night.

"If you're genuinely hungry, you'll experience authentic hunger pangs, such as belly rumbling, low energy, jitteriness, migraines, and trouble focusing."Recognizing when to pay attention to those impulses is equally crucial so that you can learn how they feel in the future. Build the columns listed below in a notepad or in the notes app on your smartphone to create your meal record:

- What you ate;
- when you ate;
- How you felt and the activities you engaged in while you ate;

Medical personnel advised that you should review your entries after a few days.

"Highlight some of the behaviors that could indicate mistaking something else, such as fatigue or being around food, for hunger."

Note the things that typically "prompt" you to eat after that. The following are examples of prevalent meal inducers:

- Watching an advertisement for something you desire to eat or entering your kitchen.
- Feeling overwhelmed, for instance, after a stressful day at work or a disagreement with a friend.
- Being offered food by a particular friend who baked you pastries.
- Depending on routines, such as drinking your preferred coffee every morning, boredom, or fatigue.

It's easier to say no to enticing food if you never have to.

This does not imply fleeing the instant someone gives you a piece of cake. It entails preparation. Do you, for example, always munch on food while watching your favorite film at home?

Choose a healthy food, such as an apple or nuts, to chew on. Or do you frequently make regular trips to the refrigerator?

Water with lemon is an excellent appetite suppressant that will urge you to wait for full meals.

"Plan for feeding impulses that you find especially difficult to resist; if you can't avoid them entirely, begin to manage them with a healthy option." If you find yourself stress-eating after work daily, keep a nutritious go-to snack on hand, such as veggies and dip or a handful of almonds.

☐ **Getting to Know Your Body**

Because life is uncertain, it is practically impossible to plan for all of your food and snacks. You'll surely come across a meal option you hadn't considered before, and it'll be up to you to decide whether or not you're truly hungry.

Following are a few techniques for monitoring your body's degree of hunger:

- Stopping and trying your best to be honest when you ask yourself if you're hungry;
- scanning your entire body from head to toe to assess your physical and mental well-being;
- Consuming food more slowly and giving your body time to signal fully.
- Diverting your attention from food by doing something different.

It's vital to be patient with yourself while you adjust to a healthy lifestyle since habits take time to form.

You'll gradually have a better understanding of your body, day by day. Make sure to acknowledge and reward yourself each time you successfully listen (but not with a cookie).

Keep in mind that you have some flexibility. "Balance is key to healthy eating, If it's your birthday, eat your cake while smiling. And with a little wiggle room, you'll be much more likely to adhere to the schedule the rest of the time. You'll be well on your way to a healthier lifestyle, whether it takes days or weeks to acclimate to listening to your body's hunger pangs.

Chapter 2

Overdesire and Overhunger: Why Your Body Is Always Hungry

I am focusing on what I would argue are the three main things driving us to overeat:

1. Overhunger

2. Overdesire

3. Eating for emotional reasons (whether consciously, in response to a craving, or on autopilot)

• Over hunger

This can be because we are using food as comfort or to distract ourselves when we have negative emotions, such as anxiety or boredom. We are not taught how to feel our feelings and manage our emotions. We also have come to believe that overeating is normal. We frequently eat throughout the day. Portions are large; it's socially acceptable to overeat.

Our brains are designed to reward us for life-preserving activities. Food provides that reward in the form of dopamine. All the cues around food—looking at it, smelling it, and tasting it—create neural pathways that remind us of how important it is for our survival to seek food again and again. Certain foods, particularly those high in sugar, are potent rewards that promote eating, even when you're not hungry. Eating foods high in sugar will trigger your brain to want to eat all the available sugary foods.

In evolutionary terms, this used to be advantageous.

It ensured that we ate food when it was available, enabling us to store energy in the body (as fat) for future needs because our food sources were sometimes scarce and unreliable. However, today, when food is widely available, this adaptation has become a liability. The more we eat sugar, the more we get the concentrated reward of dopamine hitting our brain, and the more we learn to associate the food with the reward.

The more often we do this, the stronger the corresponding neural pathway for the activity becomes.

Eventually, we get so good at it that it becomes an unconscious habit. This is why we often feel out of control and as if we are eating against our will.

As I mentioned previously, the solution to your overeating has to address all three of these components, or it will not work in the long term. I've discovered that the diet/weight loss industry and even most doctors (including obesity medicine specialists) focus on the WHAT of eating—types of foods to eat or not eat, when to eat, and how much to eat. No one seems to be focusing on the WHY of eating, which is the true underlying cause of being overweight.

So that's what I am doing with you here and in more depth: helping you understand why you are overeating, and addressing each component so that you can healthily lose body fat, for good.

Early on, we talked about various things that promote hunger, When your body is physically hungrier all the time, you will naturally want to eat more food and more often, whether it's "healthy" food or junk food.

There are probably thousands of things that can improve hunger levels, but we focused on what I view as the highest-impact pieces:

adding more protein, avoiding liquid calories, limiting sugar and refined grains, sleeping better, and eating foods rich in fiber and water.

The second main reason why we overeat is over-desire

Overdesire:

The cause of being overweight is an over-desire for food. Our desire for food is based on the healthy release of dopamine in the brain. Our desire also comes from the subtle reward healthy food provides and the satisfaction of hunger.

When we eat foods that unnaturally release a lot of dopamine, we wind up having much more desire than we need to when it comes to our food.

Our ultimate goal is to reduce the desire for overeating.

When that is gone, we will not need willpower or extra effort to resist overeating. Every day, food becomes nothing more than fuel for the body, something that is easily managed.

Our bodies are pretty good at actually telling us how much we need to eat to maintain a normal body weight when we are eating naturally occurring whole foods, and we have complex hunger and satiety signals that regulate that.

But humans are smart creatures and have figured out how to manufacture processed foods that are much more rewarding to our primitive brains—foods that evade those natural checks and balances!

If you are anything like me, you can be over-full from a big, satisfying dinner and yet still find room for dessert. It's not that you're physically hungry, it's just that the food is so damn rewarding that you eat it despite feeling satisfied. That is **over-desire**. Our brains love sugar, love fat, and love salt.

The only food found in nature that I can think of that combines both fat and sugar in a single item is breast milk, which makes sense because we want our infants to survive before they are old enough to hunt and gather their food!
Sugar, fat, and salt are things that were relatively scarce when we were evolving as hunter-gatherers, and if we came across a beehive full of honey, it was a huge jackpot.

To this day, hunter-gatherers will binge on pints of honey after braving the bees if they're lucky enough to come across a beehive. When food was scarce, binging whenever we found something calorically valuable kept our species alive.

Our modern brains are no longer living in an environment of food scarcity, but they still have this same reward mechanism to fire off pleasure-inducing neurotransmitters like dopamine, and endorphins every time we do something that historically promoted our species' survival, whether it be having sex or eating calorie-dense foods.

Food manufacturers have realized that processing and concentrating sugar and grains into easily digestible sweet, salty, and fatty bits of concentrated pleasure sets off the reward pathways in our brain much more intensely than naturally occurring foods and makes us want them more. MUCH more.

This is how food manufacturers make money, of course: by getting us to buy more of their products by making them crave-inducing. Of note, homemade baked goods are still made from processed foods like flour (a refined grain) and sugar, So don't delude yourself into thinking that homemade is exempt from the pleasure trap! So, the bottom line is, one of the greatest things you could do to start to tackle your

over-desire is to eliminate addictive processed foods (including refined grains and added sugar) from your daily diet, and save them for occasional, planned special treats.

Eating for emotional reasons

When you eat in response to emotions, it's called "emotional eating." Everyone does it sometimes. Our bodies need food to survive. It makes sense that eating lights up the reward system in the brain and makes you feel better. When emotional eating happens often and you don't have other ways to cope, it can be a problem. Although eating may feel like a way to cope in those moments, it doesn't address the true issue. If you're feeling stressed, anxious, bored, lonely, sad, or tired, food won't fix those feelings.

For some people, this cycle of turning to food to cope creates guilt and shame—more difficult feelings to navigate.

Lesson: Avoid refined grains and added sugars.

Eating a lot of high-glycemic load foods or foods high in simple carbohydrates like refined grains (e.g., white rice or flour-based foods like bread, crackers, or pasta) or sugars that are easily digested and absorbed into the bloodstream can lead to the release of constant high levels of insulin in response to the higher blood glucose level and the eventual development of insulin resistance.

Insulin resistance occurs when your body sees high levels of insulin all the time and starts to down-regulate its insulin receptors in response to the constant stimulation, ultimately making you need even higher levels of insulin to do the same job.

Insulin's job is to remove glucose from your blood and put it into cells for use as energy or turn it into fat for energy storage.

When your body's cells aren't seeing the effects of insulin working on them (whether it's because your insulin level is actually low because you haven't eaten in a while and your blood sugar is low or because you have insulin resistance and the higher levels of insulin in your blood aren't being recognized),
Your body thinks you must be low on blood sugar and therefore need to eat to get some energy, so it creates a hunger to get you to eat.
Lack of energy after eating, constant sugar cravings, and feeling hungry just an hour or two after eating are all signs of possible insulin resistance, and the way to reverse this condition is to mostly avoid eating the foods that raise insulin levels the most:

high glycemic load foods like added sugars (sweetened beverages like sweet tea, soda, or fruit juice; candy, cookies, and pastries, ice cream, honey, agave syrup, maple syrup, etc.) and foods made from refined grains (white rice, bread, crackers, pasta, tortillas, breakfast cereals, and other foods made with flour).

If you eat these foods regularly and then decide to stop, after a period of withdrawal (likely several weeks)where you may feel hungry all the time and have intense cravings for these foods, your body will eventually adjust to your new lower glycemic diet, and the lower levels of insulin required to process your food will allow your insulin receptors to start to normalize. Along with this will come sweet relief from the constant hunger you've been experiencing.

Chapter 3

Why You Give In and Eat "Bad" Food

Ever feel like you have an endless craving for all the junk food—salty, sweet, or both—that you can get your hands on?

You just can't seem to give it up and keep eating, especially during times of heavy stress. And there's certainly been plenty of stress to keep us hitting the bags of chocolate for the last several months.

"Especially when we're stressed, junk food often soothes us with the least amount of fuss and effort." "We look for sugary and fatty foods to make us feel good," says a registered dietitian. "But there are ways to get control of your food cravings instead of them controlling you."

Is "junk food" bad for you?

Junk food is food that is unhealthy for you, just as the word "junk" implies. It runs the gamut from sickly sweet (think:

cookies, candy, and cake) to heavy on saturated fats (think: fried and processed foods).

Overeating junk food can have short- and long-term consequences for your body, thanks to these ingredients.

Saturated fats `

Eating foods rich in saturated fats can increase your cholesterol levels and the amount of plaque in your blood vessels.   "diabetes,"If you have blood vessels that are stiffening and not moving blood effectively, you have a higher risk for heart disease, including heart attacks and strokes.

Sugars

Too much sugar in your diet can lead to weight gain, which is a risk factor for diabetes. Some animal studies also suggest that artificial sweeteners make our bodies resist insulin.

This may also increase the likelihood of developing prediabetes, diabetes, and heart disease.

"Most people are walking around with prediabetes, putting them at risk for developing Type 2 diabetes." Once you have `diabetes, doctors treat you as if you've already had a heart attack because the rate of heart disease is so much higher.

"All of these health issues affect all the organs, so it's important to get a handle on them."

What causes junk food and sugar cravings?

Four reasons you may be craving sweets and other junk food

- Food euphoria

Unfortunately, our bodies are hardwired to crave junk food. When you eat foods you enjoy, you stimulate the feel-good centers in your brain, triggering you to eat even more.

Especially in individuals with excess weight and obesity, the brain's reward processing system for food is like its mechanisms related to substance abuse. "Sugar makes us want to eat more sugar; fat makes us want to eat more fat," note, "Our brains are chasing that pleasurable state of food euphoria."

- Lack of sleep Studies suggest that sleep deprivation is associated with increased hunger (especially snack and sweet cravings), and you can blame it on your hormones.

Lack of sleep causes hormone shifts.

- · Ghrelin, the hunger-control hormone, increases, causing you to eat more.
- · Leptin, the appetite-suppressing hormone, decreases.
- · Cortisol, the stress hormone, may increase, stimulating your appetite.
- · Research show that sleeps deprivation causes an increase in overall hunger, which can lead to cravings for sugar, fat, or both.

3. Habit

"If it's normal for you to eat junk food, it can be hard to break that cycle." You're used to not cooking, preparing, or planning. "You eat whatever's on hand because that's what you've always done."

4. Stress

Stress, or emotional eating, really is a thing, and it's the result of both nature and nurture.

Some people find that eating helps them avoid negative thoughts and feelings. Others learned as children to use food to cope.

Hormones are also responsible, like lack of sleep, and ongoing stress causes the body to increase levels of cortisol and other hormones connected to hunger. Studies show this hormone tsunami increases appetite, along with your desire for sugary and fatty foods.

Seven ways to curb junk food cravings

These strategies can help you master your food cravings:

- **Practice mindfulness:** Try to eat and drink without distractions, "Avoid eating in the car or while watching TV or answering emails. Really focus on enjoying and tasting your food. You'll find that a few bites can satisfy your craving — and save a lot of calories."

- **Try an air fryer:** "One of the best recent inventions is the convection air fryer."

It allows you to eat things that have a fried consistency, minus the oil, "It's a healthier way to indulge."

- **Embrace meal Planning**: when you plan ahead, you empower yourself to make good decisions. "Even if you choose a food that's not healthy, it shouldn't be a problem if you plan for it by eating healthier for a couple of days before or after." Other ways to plan include stashing healthy snacks in your bag or desk and planning dinners ahead of time so your mind (and not your stomach) decides the menu.

- **Drink lots of water:** It's easy to confuse thirst cues with hunger cravings. To stay hydrated all day, keep a water bottle within reach.

- **Get a good night's sleep:** Keep those hunger hormones in check with adequate rest.

- **Manage stress:** "If you cultivate a healthy lifestyle, those cravings often go away because the body isn't responding to stress. Try meditation, exercise or reading to settle yourself down in stressful moments."

It's also OK to ask for help when you're feeling stuck. Talk with your primary care physician or a registered dietitian. That's what we're here for: to educate and empower you to make better decisions.

"We can help you choose healthier options and modifications rather than focusing on things you have to cut."

Healthy alternatives to junk food

When you make an effort to understand what flavors you do and don't like, it's easier to find healthier alternatives. A few ideas to get you started: **The same food, a different version**

- Try changing up the style of food instead of the food itself.

- Try oven-baked or air-fried versions of your favorite fried foods.

- Eat lower-sugar versions of your favorite cookies and sweets — or stick to smaller portions.

- Try pizza with 100% whole grain crust, either made from scratch or at restaurants that offer it.

- You can also make speciality crusts — made from ingredients such as cauliflower. And don't skimp on the veggies!

- Eat potatoes with the skin. The extra fiber in the potato skin helps slow digestion and keep your blood sugar in balance.

Try this instead of that if the other options do not work for you.

Figure out a great switch to keep you going.

- Have a chocolate-dipped pretzel or piece of fruit instead of an entire chocolate bar.

- In recipes, try swapping applesauce for oil or decreasing sugar by at least one-fourth.

- Next time you want a carbonated drink, opt for sparkling water without sugar or artificial sweeteners.

- Swap out white potatoes for sweet potatoes, which are lower in the glycemic index and higher in micronutrients.

- Instead of pretzels and chips, enjoy air-popped popcorn, popcorn made with extra virgin olive oil, or unsalted mixed nuts.

- Try replacing sugary treats with berries and dark chocolate (over 70%).

  Add a bit of nut butter for protein and healthy fat. Other options include berry herbal teas, frozen berries, and homemade nut balls sweetened with two to three Medjool dates.

Resisting food cravings is important if you're trying to lose weight or reduce blood pressure or cholesterol.

But there is such a thing as being too restrictive. If you're relatively healthy, at a healthy weight, and your blood pressure and blood sugar, are on point, feel free to indulge if you plan for it. "Many people eat around their cravings."

When they want something chocolatey, they eat a piece of fruit that doesn't hit the spot. Then they try an ice pop and get the same result, and it goes on.

"Just eat what you're craving, really enjoy it, and be done with it," she suggests. "That way, you'll be satisfied and won't need to go back for more."

Chapter 4

Exercise as an approach to weight loss

Exercise is essential for a healthy lifestyle. It helps keep your body and mind in shape, increases energy, and even has the potential to help prevent or manage certain diseases. The key is finding the right exercises for you and making sure you get enough of them.

It is one of the most effective approaches to losing weight. Not only does it help you burn calories and build muscle, but it also has a positive effect on your mental and emotional health. Here are some tips to help you get the most out of exercise for weight loss:

• Start slowly. Don't try to do too much, too soon. Begin with a low-intensity activity like walking and gradually increase the intensity and amount of exercise as you become fitter.

• Set realistic goals. Don't try to lose a huge amount of weight in a short amount of time.
Instead, set smaller goals that you can realistically reach. This will help you stay motivated as you go.

• Find an exercise buddy. Having someone to exercise with can make it more enjoyable and help you stay on track.

• Mix it up. If you get bored with one type of exercise, try something else. There are plenty of different exercises you can do to stay active and burn calories.

• Don't forget to rest. Exercise is important, but rest days are too. Give your body time to recover, and don't overdo it.

Exercise is an important part of any weight-loss plan. Incorporate these tips into your routine to make the most of it and get the results you want.

Cardiovascular exercises:

These are physical activities that raise your heart rate and breathing rate. This type of exercise is an essential part of any weight loss program as it helps to burn calories and increase metabolism.

It can also help to improve your cardiovascular health and reduce your risk of developing chronic health conditions such as heart disease and diabetes. Examples of cardio exercises include running, walking, cycling, swimming, rowing, stair climbing, and aerobic classes. For weight loss to be effective, you should aim for a minimum of 150 minutes of moderate-intensity cardio exercise per week or 75 minutes of vigorous-intensity cardio exercise. It is also important to combine cardio with strength training exercises to build metabolism-boosting muscle.

1. **Running**: Running is one of the best forms of cardio exercise for weight loss because it burns a large number of calories quickly. It is also an effective way to build endurance and stamina.

2. **Swimming**: Swimming is a great way to burn calories without putting strain on your joints. It helps increase your metabolism and build muscle tone.

3. **Jumping rope**: This is a great way to burn calories and get your heart rate up quickly. Jumping rope is also great for coordination and agility.

4. **Stationary Bike**: Riding a stationary bike is a great way to get your heart rate up, burn calories, and improve your aerobic capacity.

5. **Elliptical:** An elliptical is a low-impact form of exercise that is great for burning calories and improving your cardiovascular endurance.

6. **Rowing**: Rowing is an effective form of cardio that can help to burn calories and improve your fitness level.

7. **High-Intensity Interval Training (HIIT)**: HIIT is a type of exercise that involves alternating short bursts of intense activity with more extended periods of lower-intensity activity. It is a great way to burn calories and improve your fitness level.

8. **Circuit Training**: Circuit training combines strength training and cardio exercises to help you burn calories and improve your strength and endurance.

This is a practical approach to weight loss because they build muscle, and muscle burns more calories than fat.

Strength training exercises help to boost your metabolism, allowing your body to burn more calories even when you are at rest. Strength training can also help you maintain weight loss over time by helping to prevent or reduce age-related muscle loss, which can lead to an increased risk of weight gain. Additionally, strength training can help to increase your strength, coordination, and balance, which can help you to stay active and perform other types of physical activity.

Finally, strength training can help to reduce body fat, which is important for improving your overall health. When combined with regular aerobic exercise, strength training can help you achieve your weight loss goals.

Squats: Squats are a great exercise for targeting most of the major muscle groups in the body, including the quads, hamstrings, glutes, and core.

As you lower down into a squat, you're working to engage all of these muscles, making them stronger and potentially burning more calories than if you were just doing a single-muscle exercise.

Lunges: Lunges are a great strength training exercise for targeting the quads, glutes, and hamstrings.

As you lunge forward, you're working the muscles of the lower body to build strength and help burn calories.

Push-ups: Push-ups are an excellent exercise for working the chest, shoulders, and triceps. As you lower yourself, you're working to engage these muscles, helping to build strength and burn calories.

Deadlifts: Deadlifts are an excellent exercise for targeting the glutes, hamstrings, and back. As you lift the weight, you're working to engage these muscles and build strength, potentially burning more calories than if you were just doing a single-muscle exercise.

Step-Ups: Step-ups are an excellent exercise for targeting the quads, glutes, and hamstrings. As you step up onto the bench, you're working to engage these muscles and build strength, potentially burning more calories than if you were just doing a single-muscle exercise.

Pull-ups: Pull-ups are a great exercise for targeting the back, biceps, and core. As you pull yourself up, you're working to engage these muscles, helping to build strength and burn calories.

Shoulder Presses: Shoulder presses are a great exercise for targeting the deltoids and triceps. As you press the weight up, you're working to engage these muscles and build strength, potentially burning more calories than if you were just doing a single-muscle exercise.

Chest Presses: Chest presses are a great exercise for targeting the chest, triceps, and shoulders.

As you press the weight up, you're working to engage these muscles, helping to build strength and burn calories.

Lat Pull-Downs: Lat pull-downs are a great exercise for targeting the back, biceps, and shoulders. As you pull the weight down, you're working to engage these muscles, helping to build strength and burn calories.

Tricep Extensions: Tricep extensions are a great exercise for targeting the triceps.

As you extend the weight, you're working to engage these muscles and build strength, potentially burning more calories than if you were just doing a single-muscle exercise.

Bicep Curls: Bicep curls are a great exercise for targeting the biceps. As you curl the weight up, you're working to engage these muscles and build strength, potentially burning more calories than if you were just doing a single-muscle exercise.

Kettlebell Swings: Kettlebell swings are a great exercise for targeting the glutes, hamstrings, core, and shoulders. As you swing the weight up, you're working to engage these muscles, helping to build strength and burn calories.

Medicine Ball Exercises: Medicine ball exercises are a great way to target multiple muscle groups at the same time. As you throw the ball, you're working to engage the muscles of the arms, chest, core, and legs, potentially burning more calories than if you were just doing a single-muscle exercise.

Core Exercises: Core exercises are a great way to target the muscles of the core, including the abs;

Finding the right exercise program:

This is an important step in any weight loss journey. The right program should include a combination of aerobic and strength training exercises to help increase your heart rate and build muscle.

It should also include activities that you enjoy and are challenging enough to keep you motivated. Aerobic exercises, such as running, swimming, and cycling, are great for burning calories and improving cardiovascular health.

Strength training exercises, such as weight lifting, can help you build muscle and boost your metabolism.

Additionally, both types of exercise can help improve your overall physical fitness. When choosing an exercise program, it's essential to consider your available time and how often you can commit to exercising. It's also important to ensure you're comfortable with the type and intensity of exercise you're doing.

Finally, it's important to have a plan in place to track your progress. This can help you stay motivated and ensure that you're making progress towards your goals.

Tracking your progress can also help you identify any changes, you need to make to your exercise program to optimize your results. Overall, finding the right exercise program is essential for any weight loss journey.

It should include a combination of aerobic and strength training exercises that are challenging enough to keep you motivated and that you enjoy doing. Additionally, having a plan in place to track your progress is important for staying on track and making sure you're getting the results you want.

Practice Makes Perfect

The more you practice something, the easier it becomes. It takes time to etch those healthy habits into a routine. Be

Chapter 5

How to Keep Off the weight permanently

You've hit that magic number at last; now what do you do? The goal is to lose the extra weight and never find it again.

Unfortunately, only about a third of dieters are successful at maintaining their weight loss. Seasoned dieters know that keeping it off takes vigilance, and for some people, that's more difficult than the actual weight loss.

patient with yourself, and don't let all your hard work go down the tubes. Know your weaknesses and be prepared. You will be tempted by certain foods and in certain situations, but if you keep your resolve strong, you can overcome temptations. Moderation is a great approach in those tough situations. One of my favorite strategies for weight maintenance is to designate a day of the week when I let myself indulge a little.

Losing weight permanently:

This may feel like an insurmountable challenge, but it is possible to maintain the habits and behaviors that helped you lose weight.

Losing weight takes a high degree of commitment to making lifestyle changes. It would be sad to lose progress after all that hard work! Thinking ahead to how you'll maintain the weight while you're on a weight loss journey may help you focus on the long game.

The statistics on the number of people who achieve permanent weight loss are disheartening. The annual probability is less than 1% that a person will get back down to a healthy BMI level once they reach a BMI of 30 or greater. Though this study excluded bariatric patients, it does indicate that many have extreme difficulty getting to a healthy weight.

That's the bad news. The good news is that information is available on people who have lost a lot of weight and kept it off. Data and research on this group of individuals are maintained.

For some of these tips, I'm going to compare what I'm doing with some of the best tips for permanent weight loss.

These are things that have been particularly helpful in my weight management. Of course, the specific things that I find useful may also be useful to others. Those people who lose a lot of weight and keep it off have many similarities (on average)!

If you are struggling on your journey, I hope that you find tips below that help you. After the tips, I will cover some frequently asked questions that I get on the topic of weight, Having access to accurate information can be a good first step in improving your health. Happy reading!

1. Continue to self-monitor after you reach your goal weight

The journey hasn't ended once you reach your desired number on the scale. To maintain a healthy weight, continue to self-monitor your food intake in a way that does not make you feel overly restricted;

There is evidence that various dietary strategies (e.g., low fat, low carb) can work for weight loss by creating a calorie deficit.

Find one that works with your food preferences and that you can stick with long-term. I continued the self-monitoring habits that helped me while I was losing weight.

Continuing to weigh myself weekly and track my food intake.

2. Stop worrying about what others think you should or should not be doing

When major lifestyle changes are made, it seems like everyone has an opinion. Set boundaries with the people around you. Unfortunately, some people can become pushy when they see someone close to them trying to make changes. Remember that other people cannot determine your happiness or the goals that would most increase your well-being. Permit yourself to say no when someone tries to push food on you that you do not want.

3. Don't drop physical activity when you reach your goal

Find an exercise that you enjoy so that you stick with it. Regular physical activity has been shown to help people with healthy weight maintenance. The most frequently reported activity is walking.

4. Add a lot of vegetables and fruits to your meals.

Non-starchy vegetables add a lot of fiber and volume to meals for very few calories.

Adding them to (nearly) all of my meals helps me feel satisfied with the meal without gaining weight.

There is a great resource for those interested in learning about creating high-volume healthy meals that are lower in calories. Lean proteins are very filling as well. I have plain oatmeal with fresh fruit or eggs and veggies most mornings for breakfast, usually with unsweetened Greek yoghurt.

5. Limit treats with added sugar, added oils, and/or refined flour

Technically, I never set any firm rules about avoiding foods during my weight loss and current maintenance. However, I quickly learned that some food choices were wiser than others in terms of satiating effects. Certain dietary patterns seemed to be far more satisfying to me than others.

If you are aiming for permanent fat loss, it is most important to pay attention to which nutrient-rich foods are the most filling for YOU.

Whole-food carbohydrates are not necessarily the "bad guys." Highly refined carbohydrates tend to be a different story.

I generally stayed away from refined grains, flour, and added or concentrated sugars during my weight loss.

This would include not only things like cookies and cakes but also "healthier" fare like muffins, granola, and dried fruit.

I do enjoy rich desserts on my birthday and certain other special holidays.

However, I usually skip eating things like cookies, cakes, sweetened bread, and other baked goods that are largely empty calories during a typical day.

6. Limit high-calorie drinks.

I very rarely drink items like soda, sugar-sweetened teas, vitamin drinks, and juice. I don't find these items very filling, so I stick to zero-calorie beverages like water, green tea, and black coffee. In addition, I found it helpful to use some zero-calorie beverages with artificial sweeteners during my weight loss. The association of these beverages with weight loss or gain has been inconclusive.

Occasionally, I'll drink unsweetened milk, which contains more nutrients than sugar-sweetened beverages.

If I want to drink fruit, I make it into a smoothie in my food processor to retain the filling fiber that is removed from juices.

 In a survey conducted, it was found that more people want to lose weight with exercise and by making changes to their diets.

However, many people do not realize that dieting is not a one-size-fits-all solution. Because everyone has a different body, we must learn how to create customized diet plans that work best for our bodies.

Do you want to learn more about creating custom weight-loss meal plans that will give you sustained energy throughout your daily activities? Keep reading this article to learn how you can **overcome** weight loss.

Chapter 6

How to measure weight loss accurately

The fundamental issue with measuring weight loss with a scale or BMI is that neither of them takes body composition into account. The following methods of measuring weight loss are more accurate because they can differentiate between fat and muscle loss or gain.

1. Skin callipers

Skin callipers are a simple tool that measures the amount of fat that you have just under your skin (skinfold or subcutaneous fat). Measurements are taken at different places on your body and then entered into a formula that gives your body fat percentage and lean muscle mass percentage.

Regular skin fold measurements are a great way to monitor fat loss and lean muscle gain, provided the measurements are taken by someone who is experienced and trained in using skin callipers.

2. Impedance scales

Impedance scales, or body fat scales, use bioelectrical impedance to measure your body fat.
You stand on the scale barefoot, and a weak electrical current is transmitted through your body.
The scale measures the resistance to the current, which varies depending on your body composition.

Bioimpedance scales are a simple way to measure body fat, but they can be inaccurate depending on hydration changes and the quality of the scale. These scales can range from cheap supermarket options, which usually only measure the composition of your legs (then extrapolate that reading to the rest of your body), to expensive, more accurate models that have hand bars and send a current through your whole body.

3. DEXA (dual-energy x-ray absorptiometry) scanning

DEXA scanning is considered the gold standard for measuring body composition for weight loss management. It uses an X-ray beam passed over your body to measure body composition.

DEXA scanning can precisely measure body fat percentage changes as well as lean muscle mass changes.

It is relatively widely available, as it is used in most major research and high-performance sports centers.

Hydrodensitometry, air displacement plethysmography, hydrometry, computed tomography, and magnetic resonance imaging (MRI) are other highly accurate ways of measuring body composition. However, they are not easily accessible, and some may have radiation risks and be costly.

4. Body measurements

Taking body measurements is a simple way to monitor whether you are losing fat or gaining muscle. Remember that muscle is denser than fat. This means that one pound of muscle will take up less space than one pound of fat.

You can visualize this by measuring the circumference of different areas of your body. All you need is a tape measure.

Ideally, measure yourself naked or wearing tight-fitting clothes, in the following areas:

Bust: Around your chest at the nipple line

Calves: Around the largest part of each calf

Chest: Just under your bust.

Forearm: Around the largest part of the forearm (under the elbow)

Hips: Around the widest part of your hips

Thighs: Around the largest part of each thigh

Upper arm: Around the biggest part of each arm (above the elbow)

Waist: Around the smallest part of your waist, or slightly above your belly button

Although body measurements don't give you your body fat percentage, they are a simple, cheap, and easy way to monitor your body's changes.

How often should you measure your weight?

The jury is still out on this one. At the end of the day, you just have to find what works for you.

One large study of 1,042 participants found that those who weighed themselves once per week or less didn't lose weight. In contrast, those who weighed themselves six or seven times per week lost an average of 1.7%.

Daily weigh-ins may work for some people, but for others, it may be a demotivating exercise because weight loss is a slow process and weight can fluctuate on a daily basis.

For example, a review of 20 published studies concluded that repetitive self-weighing can have a negative impact on mood, anxiety, self-esteem, and eating behaviors, particularly in women and young adults.

However, it had a neutral or positive impact on people who were overweight and pursuing treatment.

If you choose to monitor your progress using skin callipers or another method of body fat measurement, you may want to stretch your measurements out to every two weeks, as body fat percentage takes a longer time to change noticeably.

Whatever method you choose, it's important that you take your measurements under the same condition each time and that you keep a record of your readings so that you can track your progress. Most importantly, try not to obsess over the numbers and the measurements. Ultimately, what matters is the changes that you can see in your body from a health, physical appearance, or fitness perspective and how you feel about yourself.

Losing weight is more complex than just watching the numbers move on a scale. It's more accurate to monitor your progress by measuring changes in your body composition.

Know what to measure for weight loss, so you don't get off track.

Your goal should be to decrease the percentage of your body fat while maintaining or increasing your lean muscle mass.

Ways to measure body composition range from body measurements and skin calliper measurements to bioelectrical impedance scales and

DEXA scanning.

Some people find that weighing in daily helps keep them accountable, while others find it more productive to measure their weight loss biweekly or even monthly.

Why your scale doesn't tell the whole story

A standard scale measures one thing: your body weight.

It's unable to differentiate between weight due to water retention, the huge meal you've just eaten, or muscle that you may have gained due to your training plan.

The following factors can influence the reading on your scale.

Your body's water weight

When we are young, our bodies are made up of about 75% water. As we get older, this percentage gradually declines until we reach around 55% water when we are elderly.

If the percentage of water in our bodies increases above the normal average and what our bodies can utilize, fluid retention happens. Consequently, our water weight and overall weight increase.

Some of the common causes of excess water weight are hormonal changes (such as premenstrual syndrome, using contraceptive pills, or pregnancy in females), high salt intake, and high carbohydrate intake. Just having a salty dinner can push your weight up the following morning.

Your body composition (how much fat and how much muscle you have)

Muscle is denser than fat, so a pound of muscle looks very different from a pound of fat. Once you are well on your way with your diet and exercise program, you should be losing fat and gaining muscle. When you step on your bathroom scale, it is unable to tell the difference between the fat that you've lost and the muscle that you've gained. So although the weight on your scale may not have dropped as much as you might have hoped, you may look very different from the way you did before you started your weight loss journey.

Your weight fluctuates.

Your weight changes throughout the day according to what you are wearing, what you eat, what you drink, how much you've sweated, and how much you've exercised.

If you don't weigh yourself at precisely the same time each day, the reading you get on your scale won't accurately reflect your weight change.

A bathroom scale can be useful, but to track your weight as accurately as possible, you need to weigh yourself at the same time each day—ideally, first thing in the morning before you've eaten or drunk anything—and under the same conditions each day.

Your body mass index (BMI)

You may have heard of the body mass index (BMI), as it's often used to define underweight, overweight, and obesity. There is a flaw with using the BMI, though.

BMI is calculated by dividing your weight (kg) by your height squared (cm).

If you are very muscular, your BMI will be on the higher side. The BMI reading will define you as overweight even though your body fat percentage could be very low.

You can't read too much into your BMI measurement, then, if you are more muscular than average.

Chapter 7

Weight Loss Challenges And How To Solve Them

Just keep in mind that to succeed in your weight loss journey, you should choose the method that works best for you, and keep a record of your progress. Consistency is key.

One of the most challenging things about losing weight can often be overcoming all the obstacles that can stand in your way. From weight-loss plateau and lack of motivation to under eating, overtraining, many challenges come hand-in-hand with trying to shed pounds and maintain a healthy weight. Overcoming them can be daunting, but it's not impossible. With the right mindset and a helping hand, you'll be on your way to reaching your goals in no time! Read on to see how to push through some common obstacles to losing weight.

1. Being Obsessed With the Number on the Scale

To lose weight *and* keep it off, you need to develop a healthy relationship with food and your body.

It means trying (it can be challenging!) not to be obsessed with the number you see on your scale. While the scale can be a helpful tool, it's important not to become obsessed with it. Remember that muscle weighs more than fat and body composition changes along with water fluctuations may result in not seeing the number change on the scale right away

Women, especially retain and lose water weight, along with bloating, throughout their menstrual cycle. This may be discouraging if you are track your progress daily.

Focusing too much on your weight may lead to unhealthy eating. Don't let the number on the scale discourage you. Instead, focus on your overall progress and how you feel physically and emotionally.

How to overcome it

- The most important thing is to focus on creating healthy lifestyles and being mindful of how your body feels.

- If you want something to measure daily, try measuring your waist with soft tapes, like the ones tailors use.
- Again, there is no need to be obsessive with this as many factors could impact this measurement.
- Remember that your weight will fluctuate daily, so using this tool may be a better option for tracking your progress over time.

2. Inappropriate Calorie Intake

To lose weight, you need to create a calorie deficit, which means burning more calories than you consume in a day. You can do this by eating healthy foods and exercising regularly.

Losing weight is hard enough, but making sure you're losing fat and not muscle can be even more challenging. Everybody is different, so you have to remember when it comes to the appropriate amount of calories for you, there's no one-size-fits-all. Underestimating the number of calories your body needs may result in the breakdown of muscle tissue for energy.

All of this may lead to serious health issues and make it even harder to lose weight in the future.

So, make sure you're aiming for the appropriate number of calories to meet your specific needs!

How to overcome it

- Depending on your weight, activity level, and goals, the number of calories you should consume each day will vary. Consult a doctor, personal trainer, or to determine your caloric intake based on your age, physical activity, and weight loss goals.

- A moderate calorie deficit is essential to promote gradual weight loss, but calories aren't the only thing that matters. Exercise, movement, and the quality of dietary choices also matter.

- You need a proper approach along with activities that help burn calories and fat to lose weight gradually and healthily. Losing weight too quickly and cutting too many calories can adversely affect your health and body.

3. Over-Exercising

Overexercising during your weight loss journey (and at any other time, for that matter) can be dangerous.

Despite this, many people are unaware of the risks associated with overtraining and still push themselves too hard.

Take lifting weights, for example.

It's a great way to become more physically fit and burn fat. Still, it is important to remember that this exercise builds muscle, which weighs more than fat.

So, you might find yourself gaining weight on your scale before losing it. But if you're patient and stick with it, you'll eventually start seeing (and feeling!) the benefits.

How to overcome it

- You need to discover the importance of listening to your body and taking days off from exercise when you need to.
- You're more likely to injure yourself if you're over-exercising, which can set your weight loss goals back.
- Remember that you won't see results overnight. Lifting weights for weight loss takes time and consistent effort.
- Small, consistent workouts are as effective as intense workouts.

4. Not Consuming Enough Protein and Fiber

When you're trying to lose weight, you might think that cutting down on calories is the way to go. However, if you're not careful, you could also cut out essential nutrients.

Protein and fiber, in particular, are two nutrients that can help you lose weight while staying healthy.

Protein enables you to maintain lean muscle mass, which is crucial for burning more calories. Fiber helps keep you feeling full so that you're less likely to overeat. Healthy fats like avocados, nuts, and fatty fish, in moderation, have a great impact on satiety. Plus, dietary fat helps with the absorption of fat-soluble vitamins.

So if you're not getting enough of these two nutrients while trying to slim down, it could be working against your goal. Also, ensure you include plenty of high-protein, high-fiber foods in your diet to help promote a healthy weight.

It can be a difficult task, especially if you don't know how to eat enough protein and fiber.

How to overcome it

- Start your day off with a high-protein breakfast. Consuming protein early in the day will help keep you feeling full. Try a full-fat, plain yoghurt or eggs for a quick and healthy start to your morning.

Fill up on fiber-rich foods at breakfast, lunch, and dinner. Veggies, fruits, whole grains, and legumes are all excellent sources of fiber.

Filling up on these foods will help prevent you from overindulging in high carbohydrate foods and sugars.

5. Not Getting Enough Sleep

Most people try to lose weight by cutting calories and increasing the amount they exercise, thinking that those are the only factors that count on their weight loss journey. Lack of sleep can counteract your effort to lose weight and may be sabotaging your diet efforts. You probably feel tired, have no energy, and feel hungry all the time if you aren't getting enough sleep.

How to overcome it

- Create a routine around your bedtime to ensure that you get enough sleep. Set a general sleep and wake time, and stick to it!
- You can help stick to a sleep schedule by setting a general time range that you eat breakfast and dinner, too.
- Begin by enjoying a book in bed before your set bedtime.

It will help you establish the routine of getting to bed on time and help you relax enough to sleep earlier.

6. Not Drinking Enough Water

Losing weight can be a complicated process, but there may be ways to make it easier. One of the ways to make it easier is by ensuring you're taking adequate water.

Many people don't drink enough water when they're trying to lose weight, making the process more complicated than it needs to be. hydration is a vital part of weight loss. If you're not drinking enough water, you may be preventing your body from losing weight.

When you hydrate properly, it allows your digestive system to effectively digest and pass on nutrients to your body, Additionally, you may be more likely to become hungry or overeat if you haven't had enough water.

How to overcome it

- Start your day with a large glass of water. It will also help you eat an adequately portioned breakfast and help you stay full until lunchtime.
- Get a gallon or water bottle. You can fill it and see how much water you are drinking throughout the day.

- How much water you need to drink will depend on your age, weight, medications you take, and exercise regime.

· The recommendation is that men drink 125 ounces (3.7 liters) of water per day and women drink 91 ounces (2.7 liters) per day. Discuss this with your doctor or a dietitian if you exercise heavily or take prescription medications.

7. Not Focusing on Nutrient Density and Quality Foods

If you're trying to lose weight, you may be making it more difficult if you're not focusing on eating high-quality foods. So, in an attempt to facilitate sustainable weight loss,
along with improving your overall health, it may be beneficial to pack your diet full of nutrient-dense foods.
It means ensuring that most of the foods you eat are packed with nutrients like vitamins, minerals, fiber, and healthy fats while being low in unhealthy ingredients like added sugar and refined grains. This approach is more effective for improving health outcomes than other methods like counting calories or cutting out certain food groups.

How to overcome it

- Balance your meals with high-quality sources of protein, healthy fats, and fiber-filled fruits, vegetables, and complex carbohydrates.
- Avoid foods containing large ingredient lists with additives like sugars, preservatives, and refined carbohydrates.
- Try and opt for fresh produce, along with minimally processed whole grains and protein.

8. You Have Unrealistic Weight-Loss Goals

Losing weight can be a difficult task, but it can be even more difficult when you set unrealistic goals for yourself.

If you want to lose weight healthily, it's important to set achievable and realistic goals. Unrealistic goals can lead to disappointment and frustration, which may cause you to give up on your weight loss journey altogether.

By setting achievable goals you can stay motivated and continue working towards your ultimate goal of losing weight.

How to overcome it

- Instead of striving for an unrealistic goal that you think you should follow, set a realistic goal that you can achieve.

- If you aren't sure what a realistic goal is for your body and individual needs, consult with a doctor or a registered dietitian. Working with a professional is a great way to understand how to set healthy, realistic goals for your weight loss journey.

Conclusion

A significant part of weight loss and management may involve restructuring the environment that promotes overeating and inactivity. The environment includes the home, the workplace, and the community (e.g., places of worship, eating places, stores, and movie theatres). Environmental factors include, the availability of foods such as fruits, vegetables, non-fat dairy products, and other foods of low energy density and high nutritional value.

Environmental restructuring emphasizes frequenting dining facilities that produce appealing foods of lower energy density and provide ample time for eating a wholesome meal rather than grabbing a candy bar or bag of chips and a soda from a vending machine. Busy lifestyles and hectic work schedules create eating habits that may contribute to a less-than-desirable eating environment, but simple changes can help to counteract these habits.

Simple changes that can modify the eating environment include:
1. Prepare meals at home and carry lunch bags
2. Learn to estimate or measure portion sizes in restaurants
3. Learn to recognize the fat content of menu items and dishes on buffet tables
4. Eliminate smoking and reduce alcohol consumption
5. Substitute low-calorie for high-calorie foods

www.ingramcontent.com/pod-product-compliance
Lightning Source LLC
Chambersburg PA
CBHW061556250726
48657CB00021B/1977